SECRETS OF A PAIN-FREE LIFE

SECRETS OF A PAIN-FREE LIFE

Recover Pain-Free Joint Motion Naturally

Dr. Stacey Raybuck Schatz DPT

ISBN-13: 9781519588210
ISBN-10: 1519588216
Library of Congress Control Number: 2016912368
CreateSpace Independent Publishing Platform
North Charleston, South Carolina

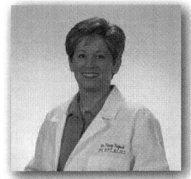

Dr. Stacey Raybuck Schatz is a Doctor of Physical Therapy and Board-Certified Orthopedic Clinical Specialist. She has thirty years of clinical practice experience, concentrated in orthopedics and sports medicine. She is the owner and director of Professional Physical Therapy and Sports Medicine in Franklin, Massachusetts, which is celebrating twenty-five years of service to the community.

While working as an emergency medical technician, she earned her undergraduate degree from the University of Massachusetts. Her post-graduate Master's and Doctorate degrees were awarded from the Institute of Health Professions, an affiliate of the Massachusetts General Hospital.

She is a trend-setter as one of the first physical therapists to obtain a Doctorate in Physical Therapy in Massachusetts.

Professionally, Dr. Raybuck Schatz is a thirty-year member of the American Physical Therapy Association, including the Massachusetts, Orthopedics, and Private Practice Sections. She has been awarded Board Certification as an Orthopedic Clinical Specialist for three consecutive ten-year terms, a rare accomplishment within the field.

Clinically, Dr. Raybuck Schatz has treated professional, elite, collegiate, amateur, and entry-level athletes in every major field, along with non-athletes of all ages, throughout her career. Having surpassed 20,000 new-patient cases, she mentors intern and resident clinicians, as well as orthopedic and sports medicine specialists. Her availability for new patients is limited, as she is dedicated to her past patients who require her expertise in musculoskeletal trauma and complex orthopedic cases of the spine and extremities.

Dr. Raybuck Schatz has authored a consumer education book—*SECRETS OF A PAIN-FREE LIFE: RECOVER PAIN-FREE JOINT MOTION, NATURALLY*—and has been a featured guest on the PT LAUNCHPAD podcast.

As the founder of the Physical Therapy Mastermind Group, now the Private Practice Collaborative of Massachusetts, Dr. Raybuck Schatz, along with other healthcare providers, promotes consumer healthcare education and legislation to ensure access to choice of provider, along with advocacy of consumer protection policies and procedures.

She is a member of the exclusive Peak Performers Mastermind Group and was a featured member on the stage at the 2016 Superconference, where Rick Harrison of the popular TV show PAWN STARS was keynote speaker.

Currently, Dr. Raybuck-Schatz travels across the nation, working as a featured motivational speaker and coach exclusively for other healthcare providers. Her clients include clinicians for professional teams, private practices, hospitals, rehabilitation facilities, and notably a doctor to the 2016 USA Olympic team.

Dr. Raybuck Schatz, has been honored with an invitation from Harvard and will be a main-stage speaker at the 2016 Harvard Business School's Expert Forum.

Dedication

This book is dedicated to *you*. The purpose of this book is to provide you with the tools and information to give you a better understanding of your options for treatment when you have pain with movement from conditions such as arthritis.

"An educated consumer has been a goal with patient care and is my vision for writing this book."

Read the book and use it. Share it with people you want to help.

Keep Moving Through Life,

Dr. Stacey Raybuck Schatz, PT, DPT, MS, OCS
Doctor of Physical Therapy
Board-Certified Owner Clinical Specialist

Table of Contents

In high school, I was the captain of the gymnastics team. During my floor routine a tumbling pass went wrong, and I watched in horror as my right elbow dislocated and bent- the wrong way.

I was initially under the care of a soon-to-be-retired orthopedic doctor who told me that my arm was essentially disabled, that he didn't "believe in physical therapy" and that I would be unable to ever use it again. And for quite a few months, I couldn't.

Fortunately, a family friend insisted I go for a second opinion to the chief of hand surgery at Mass. General Hospital. The surgeon was obviously appalled at my condition and spent much of that morning reviewing my case and films, taking pictures of my arm and movement, and then escorting me to the physical therapy department. I spent many months in that department, before and after the numerous surgeries it took to restore function of my arm. This surgeon's view was that he could repair the internal damage, but the real key was from the physical therapist who could restore my ability to use my arm, and to return to a normal life.

While I don't have a "perfect arm", I do have nearly full use of it, and I went on to become a doctor of physical therapy.

I have now been practicing for 30 years, and my clinic, Professional Physical Therapy and Sports Medicine has celebrated 25 years of service in Franklin. I have now been part of the recovery and rehabilitation process for over 20,000 patients, an honor and privilege.

Over the years, I have tried to spend "extra" time with patients, explaining and educating them about the nature of the diagnosis, options for treatment, and tips and advice. I use analogies often, and I seek to put complex medical concepts into easily understood terms. As a result, I have had patients encourage me to write a book. It only took 30 years, but here it is!

I hope that you will pick up some tips, helpful explanations, and information that will answer questions you might have. What follows are the more common questions I get asked, usually by people who have little prior experience with physical therapy. If you have never had physical therapy before, don't worry! At Professional Physical Therapy and Sports Medicine we make therapy enjoyable and rewarding. This book is meant to be a companion on your journey. Enjoy it. Pass it along to others who are in pain. Just like the family friend who steered me to a better path of recovery, please do the same for those in your life.

We are proud that we rely on obtaining new patients through the recommendations from our past and current patients. We greatly appreciate your referrals. Please share this book with others, or request a free copy to share.

Keep moving through life,
Dr. Stacey Raybuck Schatz
Owner
Professional Physical Therapy and Sports Medicine
620 Old West Central St
Franklin, Mass 02038
508-528-6100
www.ProPTinc.com

Fast Pain Relief: How Can I Get Rid of Pain Quickly?

HEAT OR ICE, MEDICATIONS, INJECTIONS, SURGERY

When you are experiencing significant pain in your joints, you have some options for pain relief—even if the relief is temporary:

- Cold packs—recommended for significantly irritated or swollen areas, cramps, and for high levels of pain such as within the first few days of an injury or after surgery. Frozen bags of peas or corn, ice cubes in a baggie, or flexible gel packs work well.

  Hint: Put the ice pack in a pillow case and apply to the painful area for twenty minutes at a time.

  Warning: Do not apply ice packs directly to the skin—every year I see cases of frostbite as a result of not using any skin protection.

- Hot packs—usually for muscle aches, or tight areas, such as morning stiffness. Enjoy a bath, shower, hot tub, herbal microwave pack, or heating pad for twenty minutes at a time.

  Hint: Warm water in a double-sealed gallon sized baggie inside of a pillowcase works well.

  Warning: Do not use hot water and do not use heating pads through the night. One of the most common accidental injuries I see is from patients who fall asleep with a heating pad and sustain a burn.

- Ointments/creams—BENGAY, Aspercreme, Biofreeze, Tiger Balm

  Hint: Unlikely to help much, but an option if you are in pain and want to try something extra. Clinically, BioFlex is popular and is available only in health professional offices. BENGAY, Aspercreme, and Tiger Balm can all be purchased at your local drugstore.

- Massage—Therapeutic, Deep Tissue, Self-massage with stick massagers and foam rollers.

  Hint: If your painful area is very tender to touch, do not pursue massage. Wait until you can perform self-massage without pain. Start with therapeutic or light/relaxation massage before deep tissue work.

- Medications—anti-inflammatories, analgesics, narcotics

  Hint: Physical therapists do not currently prescribe medications and therefore do not provide medical advice regarding pharmaceuticals. Talk openly with your pharmacist and doctor about what you are taking for pain, including the quantity of pills you are taking.

  Warning: Do not mistake over-the-counter products as "safe." The most common thing I see patients do wrong when seeking pain relief is the overuse of pain medications, including over-the-counter pills such as ibuprofen (Advil, Motrin). It is a daily occurrence that patients report taking "handfuls" of pills to manage pain, often for long periods of time. You do not want to trade one problem for another. Seek medical advice if this sounds like you.

  Cortisone injections are another option sometimes offered for joint pain. If injected at the right spot, cortisone injections may provide relief, but they carry a risk of complications and may cause deterioration of the cartilage within a joint. These shots are often limited in frequency as a result.

Hint: I usually present the following to my patients: Cortisone is an aggressive medication. So aggressive that it can actually damage the tissues in an effort to help. I advise delaying the option of cortisone injections when possible, as they may not help long-term.

- The surgical option—why not do surgery right away and just clean it out and fix it up? I know many people who are in pain are hopeful that there's a quick and permanent fix because arthroscopic procedures are so commonplace in orthopedics and incisions are tiny.

Hint: Many patients minimize the extent of surgical procedures, side effects, recovery and rehab needed afterwards. It is best practice to try conservative options before undergoing surgery.

Even patients who require orthopedic surgery are often referred for a course of preoperative rehabilitation physical therapy, referred to as prehab, prior to surgery. What we observe is that the better patients go into surgery, the better they come out. The length of recovery and rehab is often shortened when patients have undergone rehab prior to surgery. An added advantage is that patients are able to develop a rapport with their physical therapist ahead of time and report feeling more comfortable working with someone they know, like, and trust throughout the process.

RICE RULE

For acute injuries and flair-ups, start with RICE: Rest, Ice, Compression, and Elevation:

| Rest: | Rest and protect the area by taking it easy and avoiding any activity that may be causing your pain and soreness. |
| Ice: | Cold will reduce pain and swelling. |

| Compression: | Compression by lightly—not tightly, wrapping the injured or sore area with an elastic bandage or neoprene support can reduce pain and swelling. |
| Elevation: | Elevate the injured or sore area on pillows. Try to keep the area at or above the level of your heart to minimize swelling. Continuing with gentle movement through the available range of pain-free motion is advised to prevent the development of stiffness. |

TREATING SYMPTOMS VERSUS THE CAUSE

Temporary options for pain relief may alleviate the problem in the short term and get things moving in the right direction, but they do not address the cause of the problem. They may even have potential side effects and complications and may not work at all. Medications such as analgesic and narcotics, anti-inflammatories, and muscle relaxers may help calm symptoms, but they do not cure. It is like taking medications for cold or allergy symptom relief, not curing the cold or allergy. This is not like taking antibiotics to cure an infection. Keep this in mind when you use these medications.

> Hint: Controlling pain with medications is temporary. It will provide relief for the symptoms. Medication is not a cure.

There are many things to consider when choosing options for pain relief. Ask yourself: Is this option focused on the SYMPTOM ONLY or on the CAUSE of the problem? For example, when you have a blocked sink and use a chemical to open up the drain, it may create an opening, even a small one, for the passage of water, or it may do nothing, especially for a significant blockage. The chemicals can be dangerous and can damage pipes over time if used often. If unsuccessful, it is often necessary to have the blockage manually or mechanically removed.

Hint: With joint pain, treating the symptom is similar to using chemicals on a plugged drain. It may relieve some of the problem, but is not likely to fix it or prevent it from returning.

TAKEAWAYS from CHAPTER 1

- Treating the SYMPTOMS with pain-relieving measures is OK in the short term, but it does not address the CAUSE of the problem.
- Try conservative treatments first—fewer medications, injections, and less surgery. Physical therapy is conservative care. At Professional Physical Therapy we strive to see emergency patients within 48 hours. If you need to be seen quickly, call the office at 508-528-6100. Let the receptionist know you need an appointment as soon as possible.
- RICE Rule: Rest, Ice, Compression, and Elevation for acute injuries.

Right and Wrong Ways to Recover Pain-Free Motion

There are a few principles to keep in mind when recovering or rehabilitating painful motion. Let's start with a few of the most common ones:

PHASES OF HEALING AND RECOVERY

First, recovery is dictated by the principles of healing. Tissues go through stages or phases of healing like children go through levels of development or learning. During each phase, the right application of the right treatment will be well received by the tissues and enhance recovery. Conversely, the wrong application of the wrong treatment at the wrong phase can delay or prevent recovery. Rehabilitation that is overly cautious delays progress. Rehabilitation that is overly aggressive can lead to increased pain and inflammation, thereby slowing the healing process. Ideally, recovery will be progressive, consistent, and steadily adjusted to the healing phases of the tissues.

Inflammation/Acute Phase

Following injury (and surgery), there are chemical reactions in the body that cause inflammation that leads to swelling, redness, increased temperature, loss of function, and high levels of pain. This is the time when pain medications are most used and abused. This phase can last about one to two weeks. This is why RICE is needed—rest, ice, compression, and elevation.

Thoughts on pain medication: Ongoing research suggests that use of pain medications over time actually makes you feel pain MORE, therefore increasing the likelihood you will "need" more pain medication. The quicker you are able to wean yourself off pain medication, the better.

Thoughts on smoking: We all know that smoking is unhealthy. However, did you know that smokers heal approximately 50 percent slower than nonsmokers? If you smoke, and wonder why it takes you longer to heal than others, this is a significant factor. Taking it further, if you heal slower, perhaps you feel pain longer, which may put you at higher risk to potentially abuse pain medications.

RULE: Use more RICE and less VICE: Rest, Ice, Compression, and Elevation for pain and inflammation. Use fewer prescription and over-the-counter medications, and avoid alcohol, tobacco, and illicit substances.

Repair/Subacute Phase

During this phase, the tissues are attempting to repair and heal. Early in the healing process, the healing tissue is fragile and vulnerable. Gentle and progressive increases in motion and function are important. Too little movement, through prolonged immobilization, leads to scar tissue and loss of functional movement. Too aggressive movement re-injures the tissue and slows the healing process. This phase is critical, and can make or break your recovery and rehabilitation after injury or surgery. This is the most common time frame when patients start physical therapy and generally lasts from one week to three months after injury/surgery.

Hint: This is the danger zone of recovery. Here are two extremes I see daily in my practice:

1. Overly Cautious: These patients tend to be "afraid" to do anything wrong and do nothing at all. They are led by

fear of pain and fear of damaging tissues; they "baby" their injured area even after being medically advised against it. These patients often delay onset of physical therapy out of fear and resist instructions to discontinue pain medications, slings, crutches, braces, etc. By the time these patients start physical therapy, they are behind the norm for healing and function recovery and are at higher risk for adhesions/scar tissue and permanent loss of motion and function. Remedy includes focus on patient education, explaining the healing process, advising on "normal" and "abnormal" levels of pain, and encouragement to conquer fear. These patients often do very well once this is carefully explained by an experienced clinician. Once in treatment, their course of rehabilitation progress can be described as consistent and steady.

2. Overly Aggressive: These patients tend to be a "type A" over-achievers. They are led by the desire to heal faster than others, and to resume their activity level too quickly. They generally report doing more than advised and perceive this to be a good thing. "I was able to get rid of the sling, crutches, and brace in two days instead of two weeks"; "I can't wait two more weeks to start running again, I need to start now"; "It may take others three months to recover, but I am going to do it one month." These patients occasionally think they do not need physical therapy, that they can "do it by themselves." Early on, these patients may appear to be doing better than the norm, but their success generally does not last. They have a tendency to experience many significant setbacks, sometimes damaging surgically repaired tissues. Remedy includes focus on patient education, explaining the healing process and time frames, advising on risks/complications of overloading fragile tissues, and suggesting alternative outlets for safe activities. I refer to these patients of mine as being on a "short leash"— needing to be held back from sprints and crashes.

There is much to be said for "slow and steady wins the race." The person who benefits most from physical therapy is YOU, the patient. As a physical therapist I am less concerned with how long it takes you to finish the race as I am with preparation and crossing the finish line.

Rule: You cannot speed up the natural healing process, but you can screw it up. Slow and steady does prevail over fast and furious.

Remodeling Phase

Within the time frame of weeks and months after injury and surgery, the tissues go through a maturing phase in which they remodel and strengthen. This is the time frame when progressive attention to full motion and strength recovery is completed. At this stage, the tissues are more "solid." As full function and a high level of activity return, treatment requires the steady advancing of goals and challenges. In physical therapy, this is often the phase where patients are transitioning back to normal and weaning appointments in preparation for graduation from treatment.

CONSERVATIVE VERSUS ACCELERATED REHABILITATION

So why are recovery and rehab sometimes accelerated? Younger, healthier people heal faster. As a result, recovery and rehab can sometimes be accelerated. This is one reason why younger, athletic patients are on more accelerated programs. Patients often ask how athletes, especially professional athletes, recover so quickly. This, along with the availability for daily rehab and on-site training, are helpful factors. Additionally, professional-level teams such as the New England Patriots, Red Sox, Bruins, and Celtics retain specialized medical staff who specialize in the treatment of young, healthy, elite-level athletes. Their full-time job is to be athletes. These are highly motivated, dedicated patients whose careers and livelihoods are on the line. Older adults, especially those with other medical conditions or who smoke or don't take excellent care of themselves, will recover and rehab more slowly.

Also, newer surgical procedures lend themselves to a more conservative approach. The truth is that until long-term outcomes have been studied, we simply do not always know what to expect. The risks may outweigh the benefits; therefore until they are studied, the default is to proceed slowly. There are not always posted "speed limits" in rehabilitation, but as research advances, we narrow the range. Proceeding with caution is always the better, more informed approach.

If you want to improve your recovery of pain-free motion, do not smoke, and do eat healthy, address medical and health conditions quickly, and be a good patient. That means adhering to instructions, home programs, and appointments, and communicating your questions and concerns in a timely manner.

NO PAIN, NO GAIN: TRUTH OR FICTION?

"No pain, no gain" is a fallacy. If you are doing something that significantly increases pain, you need to stop and reassess. Recovery and rehab is not completely pain-free. Usually there is some discomfort involved at some stages in the process. There should be a reason why you experience increased discomfort. For example, it is common for patients to have increased discomfort during manual therapy, joint mobilization, or stretching of tight tissues. This should be temporary and relieved quickly. There is normal, new exercise soreness that you may experience as if you just started a new exercise program at the gym.

Hint: Balance the need for exercise with the need to exercise common sense.

Advice I give to my patients: "You want to talk nicely to the tissues for slow, steady progress. Don't beat them into submission."

There are many factors involved that affect the healing stages, level of progressions with recovery and rehab, accelerated results, and type of soreness, discomfort, or pain being experienced. This is why you need someone with expertise in these areas to guide you. This is what physical therapists do every day.

TAKEAWAYS from CHAPTER 2

- There are progressive stages of tissue healing, and this is an important factor for determining that the right treatment is applied at the right time. Expertise with recovery progress is crucial. At Professional Physical Therapy we have taken care of over 20,000 patients in 25 years.
- Younger, healthier, motivated patients heal faster and allow for accelerated results. Older, sicker, noncompliant patients do not progress as fast or achieve optimal results.
- Discomfort with new activity during rehab is normal, but there is no truth to "No Pain, No Gain."

3

Will Physical Therapy Help or Not?

WILL PHYSICAL THERAPY HELP?

The short answer is you don't know, and I don't know either. The main thing I want you to take away from this chapter is this:

WHAT TO DO FIRST

Try physical therapy first—before resorting to medications and injections that are full of side effects, before trying expensive and unproven as-seen-on TV gimmicks, and before undergoing drastic and permanent surgery.

Physical therapy is natural, more holistic, and focused on keeping you moving through life. If your physician does not offer a referral to physical therapy as a first option, ask them about it yourself. Sometimes physicians, especially primary care physicians, focus more on prescribing medications for symptoms and are not well-informed about physical therapy. A delay in referral to physical therapy often results in prolonged symptoms and recovery. Be your own advocate and an ambassador to your own health.

X-RAYS/MRI: NECESSARY OR NOT?

Do you need x-rays and/or MRI first? There are benefits with certain conditions to having films completed first. If your physician believes your condition requires that x-rays and/or MRI are necessary, he or she will discuss this with you. In most cases, preliminary studies are not necessary and are not helpful. X-rays show bones. They don't show soft tissue structures like tendons, ligaments, cartilage, and muscle. Remember that the body shows its age, both inside and outside. Just as we get gray hair and wrinkles on the outside as we age, the body inside shows its age with skeletal wear and tear. It is normal, therefore, to see various changes on films as we age. This is often not at all correlated with your symptoms, so I advise my patients that we don't treat x-rays and MRIs, we treat people. If your physical therapist determines that additional studies are needed, he or she will advise you and your physician so that this can be addressed. It is true that many insurance plans will not authorize payment for studies such as MRIs without trying conservative care such as physical therapy first.

WHOM TO CALL FIRST?

Can you just decide to see a PT first before seeing my doctor? Depending on your insurance coverage, a prescription or referral order form from your doctor and/or an insurance referral may be required. Certain states require a prescription from your physician. Your physician may require you to be seen in the office first in order to obtain this. It is our preference that when you are having a condition that you have never had before or are having symptoms significantly worse or without known cause, you consult first with your doctor to rule out any medical pathology. Your primary care physician may help to diagnose the cause of the problem and direct you in an appropriate direction. I have seen cases of unspecified left arm pain that were symptoms of cardiac pathology but were assumed to be coming from the shoulder by the patient. Medical screening by your primary care physician can help to screen and evaluate problems such as this.

TAKEAWAYS from CHAPTER 3

- Physical therapy treatment is considered conservative, natural, and holistic as opposed to medications, injections, and surgery
- TRY PHYSICAL THERAPY FIRST—before more aggressive, invasive, and side-effect laden treatments.
- Findings on x-rays and MRIs do not always correlate with symptoms, as the body shows its age on the inside as well as the outside.
- Medical screening by your doctor is a good first step for new problems, or for symptoms that appear suddenly and without cause. If this is a recurring problem, or one you have discussed with your doctor in the past, they may choose to refer you directly, without being seen in their office. They can fax a PT order directly to the office at 508-528-6304.
- Insurance and state requirements may mandate prescription for PT, and/or an insurance referral form from your doctor. We have 25 years of experience with insurance requirements and can help you with this. Call the receptionist at 508-528-6100 with your insurance questions, and she can advise/direct you accordingly.

4

Who Are the Movement Experts?

Aren't physical therapists, personal trainers, massage therapists, and chiropractors all the same thing? Absolutely not. This is a big misconception among the public, and physical therapy has not been well-branded by us. The profession of physical therapy first developed as a special medical unit of the army for rehabilitation of soldiers and then patients with polio. It separated from the American Medical Association in the 1950s and has continued to grow significantly since then. Physical therapists utilize a scientific basis for services while ensuring patient safety and applying evidence to provide efficient and effective care.

Personal trainers are NOT healthcare providers and are NOT licensed to perform any type of rehabilitation. Their role is as a fitness professional for the general healthy population, and they require medical clearance by a medical professional for participation. The initials PT after someone's name must mean physical therapist. Personal trainers are not allowed to use the initials PT after their name. Physical therapists often refer our graduating patients from physical therapy to personal trainers for continued fitness and exercise.

MASSAGE THERAPISTS

Massage therapy is the manual manipulation of soft tissues to enhance relaxation and for temporary pain relief. Massage therapists are NOT medical providers and cannot diagnose or treat medical issues. Massage therapy can be beneficial for relieving tight muscles and tension. Physical therapists often refer patients to massage therapists for relief of painfully tight soft tissues as an adjunct to physical therapy care.

CHIROPRACTORS

Chiropractic did NOT develop within the medical model and has remained outside mainstream medicine. While less controversial than in the past, research has documented that fraud, abuse, and quackery are prevalent in chiropractic. In my experience, chiropractic manipulation for general back pain can be beneficial for short-term relief. Attempts by chiropractors to diagnose and treat other conditions is much more controversial, along with seemingly never-ending plans of care involving unnecessary "maintenance visits."

TAKEAWAYS from CHAPTER 4

- Physical therapy started as a special medical unit of the army, separating from the American Medical Association in the 1950s.
- Personal trainers, massage therapists, and chiropractors are NOT physical therapists and can NOT perform physical therapy.

5

Control Your Destiny

My (fill in the blank—mother...father...) had bad (fill in the blank—knees...hips...): does this mean I am destined to have it, too? This is one of the most common questions I hear from patients. The most important point to keep in mind while reading this is that your architecture is somewhat genetic and you have little control over it. For example, you cannot control how tall you are, and it is more than likely that your overall build will resemble that of your parents. Even our posture and walking is affected by how our parents stood and walked. What you do with what you are given is important. If you are stiff or have poor flexibility, do you try to work extra hard on it or do you avoid stretching and flexibility activities because it is difficult for you?

We lose flexibility, strength, and endurance as we age, so activities that encourage these become increasingly more important. One of the most common recommendations made for patients is yoga. Yoga is a great way to work on flexibility, posture, balance, and core strength. The key to success is to choose an appropriate level of yoga. Do some research on what is best for you. Good instructors will help you modify positions and movement patterns as needed.

Arthritis is among the most common maladies in adults. It is estimated that you have a 40 percent likelihood of having knee arthritis if one of your parents had it. You have approximately a 65 percent likelihood of inheriting arthritis in hands and hips.

Joint replacements are at the top of the list of most frequently performed surgeries. Based on this information alone, it is more likely than not that you will experience it.

ARE MY OLD SPORTS INJURIES CATCHING UP WITH ME?

Damage to a joint can contribute to the development of arthritis in that joint later on in life. An active lifestyle has more advantages than disadvantages. One of those disadvantages, however, is that injuries may result from an active lifestyle. In the past when injuries occurred on the field or on the court, players were told by coaches to run it off or shake it off. As a result, many athletes played through injuries, not allowing for proper recovery or rehabilitation. We have seen a shift recently in the assessment and evaluation of injuries immediately at the time of the injury. The current controversy with concussion management is an example of how injury management continues to improve. Because of poor injury care years ago, we have seen arthritis develop or worsen in joints later on and often even earlier in life.

There is more attention to prevention, conditioning, training, and injury management now than in the past. Proper diagnosis, recovery, and rehab are well recognized as necessary today. Future generations will hopefully avoid much of the pain and stiffness from old injuries progressing to arthritis as they age.

Speaking of age, can you be too old to recover? The short answer is no. We all know eighty- and ninety-year-olds who act more like sixty-year-olds, and vice-versa. Overall, health and genetics play a part, but YOU have control as well. Healthful eating, staying physically and mentally fit, avoiding over indulgence in food and drink, and not smoking improve your chances of better health, and therefore a healthy and successful recovery.

AGE, WEIGHT, OUT OF SHAPE

The risk of developing many types of arthritis increases with age and is more common in women.

What about weight and being out of shape? Excess weight can contribute to both the onset and progression of knee and hip arthritis. For people who are overweight and out of shape, it is very important that they rely on a physical therapist to guide them in rehab and on starting new exercise routines. Being overweight does put additional stress on weight-bearing joints such as hips and knees. But while losing excess weight is highly desirable, it does not reverse joint damage. It can, however, alleviate additional stress and thus prevent or delay further damage. An analogy I often use with my patients is that your joints are like tires on your car; if you put too much pressure on them through excess weight, they will wear out faster. Likewise, if you drive on pothole-ridden roads, your tires will sustain more damage. If you engage in high-impact activities, your joints will likely wear out faster.

You do not have to be an athlete to be in good physical shape. Many people are active doing other things. Walking, gardening, home improvement projects, even cooking and cleaning, can be good forms of activity. Physical therapy programs encourage healthy activity. It is not about becoming a weight lifter or running a marathon. Depending on your lifestyle, health, and activity level, the physical therapist will customize appropriate levels of exercise and rehab for your success and will modify your program for your needs. Keep in mind that we often work with people who are medically deconditioned after serious injuries or illness and have expertise working with a wide variety of ages and disabilities.

TAKEAWAYS from CHAPTER 5

- You may be predisposed to various conditions genetically, but what you do to minimize and manage them controls your destiny and is most important.
- Maintaining flexibility, strength, endurance, and an active life style is best.

- Prevent injury with proper conditioning and take injuries seriously. Seek proper diagnosis and treatment, including physical therapy, to prevent long-term complications.
- Excess weight wears out joints faster.
- Movement is needed for a healthy and active lifestyle. You do not have to go the gym; just be active.

6

Common Misconceptions about Physical Therapy

1. It takes too much time. Typical physical therapy sessions range from thirty to sixty minutes per session. The average length of our plan of care at Professional Physical Therapy & Sports Medicine is ten to eleven visits. The reason that our plans of care are so much less than others is our focus on patient education, home programs, results-based treatments, and transitioning to independence. One reason that I advise people to become well-educated on the cause of their symptoms is so they can better address problems earlier and more efficiently. The longer you wait, the worse it may get and the longer it will take. Patients who have had surgical procedures or traumatic injuries generally require more sessions. Along with the time it takes, let me advise you to be aware of your options regarding appointment times. At Professional Physical Therapy, we offer early morning and later evening appointments, and Saturday appointments may be available.

2. It is too expensive. First, keep in mind the cost of medications, doctor visits, MRIs, x-rays, surgeries, and anything else you are using to reduce symptoms. What is the problem costing you in terms of lost time at work, with your family, and/or activities? Medical insurance plans cover physical therapy services. The number of visits, length of time, and requirements for coverage vary by company.

Sometimes deductibles, co-payments, or coinsurance is required. We are required to obtain your financial portion. There are some things we are able to do to help with the cost of visits, and we can work out a payment plan with you. Focusing on home programs and transitioning away from clinic services to independent programs is another way we try to keep costs down, along with attention to maximizing the value of your visits.

3. Maybe it will go away by itself. Maybe, but ask yourself a couple of questions first. How long has it been there? How bad is it? If it has been there for more than two to three weeks and/or is above a mild pain level, here is the advice I give to my patients on when to call me: Is it getting more intense, is it lasting longer, are episodes increasing in frequency? If so, it is time to be seen. The number one mistake people make with their pain is ignoring it when it's mild. Address it early when it's mild and easier to treat.

4. Maybe I will find a magic cure. Unfortunately, there are many people trying to make money by selling gimmicks to people in pain. Every couple of months there is a new infomercial, commercial, or advertisement for a new product that will magically make your pain and your money disappear. Don't be a victim of these scams. A placebo effect can be as high as 25 to 30 percent. This means that people convince themselves that something is working even when it is really not.

Millions of dollars are wasted every year on such gimmicks. Spend your money wisely on things that have proven results.

7

How to Measure Success with Treatment

When experiencing discomfort, it is important to understand the difference between exercise-related muscle soreness and pain. Here are some easy ways to tell the difference.

Pain is usually more intense than discomfort or soreness. People often describe pain as being sharp, stabbing, or throbbing, and something that interferes with activities like sleeping, working, walking, housework, etc. On a 0–10 pain scale, pain perception is generally 4 and above. Pain does not have to be constant. It may only occur with certain positions or activities. Pain is often what leads people to seek treatment quickly.

Discomfort is a lower intensity level of pain. People often describe discomfort as being dull, aching, and annoying. It does not stop them from an activity but makes the activity or position uncomfortable, either during or after. On a 0–10 scale, discomfort is generally below 4. Discomfort at some level can be constant in chronic conditions. Discomfort is often ignored by people for quite a while before seeking treatment.

Soreness and discomfort are basically the same thing, but are described differently based on cause. Soreness is usually described as discomfort resulting from exercise or a new activity. In the rehabilitation environment, some post exercise soreness is normal.

QUANTIFY AND QUALIFY

So why is all of this important? Because it is one of the things you will be asked about during your initial evaluation and on subsequent treatment sessions. I ask my patients to rate their pain on a 0–10 scale, where 0 is no pain and 10 is the worst imaginable pain. To avoid exaggeration of pain, I also tell my patients that if they are experiencing 10 out of 10 pain on a constant level, I will call the ambulance and send them to the emergency room. I want to know the pain number at its best, worst, and the usual level along with what positions, activities, and times of day affect it.

For example, here is a common patient report. "I have 0 out of 10 pain when I am sitting and resting. It is up to a 3 out of 10 when I reach overhead to get a cup out of the cabinet. It spikes to a 5 out of 10 when I reach behind to put on my coat or seatbelt. The worst pain is a 7 out of 10 when I lie on my side, and it wakes me up at night if I roll over on it."

Along with the positions and activities, you'll be asked about what you have tried on your own to decrease symptoms and how that has worked. For example, here is a common patient report: "I take two anti-inflammatory pills every four hours during the day to keep pain level at 3 out of 10 instead of 5 out of 10. When it is really bad, I use ice, and that helps. I have been using ice three times a day the past week."

The reason I am spending more time on this is that it is very important for you to accurately describe and quantify your symptoms to your medical providers for proper diagnosis and treatment and to measure the results of treatment. As I prescribe a course of treatment, I ask my patients to give updated numbers on pain. I generally ask for an overall percentage of improvement in symptoms as well. Two ways that success with treatment is measured is by a reduction in pain numbers and by reports of improvement as an overall percentage.

EVALUATE AND REEVALUATE

Throughout the course of treatment, I will ask my patient what percentage better they are now compared with when we started the therapy. If we go back to our previous examples, the patient may return the next visit reporting the ability to decrease medication usage to one pill every four hours and a 2 out of 10 pain with reaching in the cabinet instead of 3 out of 10, and 4 out of 10 with sleeping instead of 6 out of 10. Furthermore, the patient may report improvements in motion and strength based on activities, leading to a report of 50 percent overall improvement in symptoms since the onset of treatment. One key to measuring the success of treatment is your detailed feedback on the reduction of pain intensity, frequency, and duration. Another way to measure success with treatment is by repeating measurements during the course of treatment. For example, we use a tool called a goniometer to measure the range of motion of many joints. When you are undergoing rehab for limitations in joint motions, repeated measurements will be taken to gauge progress. Some motions may improve faster than others, and your program may need to be modified accordingly.

The goals for motion achievement should be discussed during your program. For example, should you expect your left knee range of motion to equal that of the right, or will it be close but not equal? With some surgical procedures a full range of motion may not be achievable. Our goal is to maximize the motion achievable. I like for my patients to know their numbers. For example, if knee flexion, was 80 degrees initially and our goal is 120 degrees, it is motivating to see the hard work pay off as it progresses to 90 degrees, 100 degrees, and up as we remeasure during visits.

It is not just about the numbers, though; it's also about function. Sitting in a chair with your feet on the ground requires approximately 90 degrees of knee bending, walking upstairs normally 95 to 100 degrees, and downstairs 105 to 110 degrees. Kneeling or squatting down to the floor require even more. Other measurements taken for monitoring progress include strength, balance, walking, and swelling. Physical therapists assess and address the quality of your movements, postures, and functions as well. During our evaluation, reevaluation, and discharge reporting, we update all of this information and document it in your medical record. A copy of these reports are sent to the physician you specify.

TAKEAWAYS from CHAPTER 7

- Pain can be described in different ways—"soreness" is usually less intense than "discomfort," which is less intense than "pain."
- Be prepared to describe your pain level on a 0–10 scale and to report what positions and activities affect your pain level.
- Measuring success with treatment is important. Be prepared to report on changes in pain levels with activities after treatment and between sessions. 0–10 pain scales and percentage better are two common things you will be asked.
- Physical therapists repeat measurements of swelling, motion, strength, walking pattern, etc., along with specific tasks and overall function during the course of treatment.
- Physical therapists write evaluations, reevaluations, and discharge reports during the course of care, and copies are sent to keep your referring physician updated.

8

How to Keep It Away

How can I prevent the problem from returning or worsening? Arthritis is a long-term condition, without a cure. There are treatments to manage it. What is important to remember is that managing pain, stiffness, and swelling improves motion and flexibility. Maintaining a healthy weight and exercise go a long way toward living a pain-free lifestyle.

Be aware of changes in symptoms and/or activities and don't minimize the significance of these changes. Pay attention to the frequency, duration, and intensity of symptoms. Address problems early when symptoms are less severe and easier to treat.

Engage in some level of activity or exercise you like, plus a little of something you need like stretching, strength training, posture, and balance. Change up your activity routine by adding variety and challenging yourself a little.

Consult with a physical therapist and become involved in your treatment. Learn ways to manage your symptoms for the long term. When you graduate from physical therapy, ask the therapist for the top three exercises for you to do to prevent the problem from occurring, and do them!

Eat healthy, lose excess weight, stop smoking, and have a positive attitude. Studies demonstrate that a positive outlook boosts the immune system and increases ability to handle pain. For more information, including upcoming books, free exam days, and free workshops please check our website www.proptinc.com and add your name to our monthly newsletter list.

David Anderson

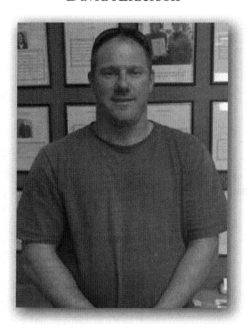

"When I came to physical therapy I had pinched a C-8 nerve in my neck. I had extreme pain and numbness down my left arm. My left arm had about 50 percent strength, and my coordination was way off. Along with not being able to work, I had a lot of trouble finding a comfortable position to sleep. Within the first couple of weeks I could feel the pain working its way back up my arm, until six weeks later I'm pain-free. I have full strength and mobility. I am very satisfied with my experience here at Professional PT. All the staff members were professional and knowledgeable."

—David Anderson

MY PHYSICAL THERAPY STORY

Walter Eaton

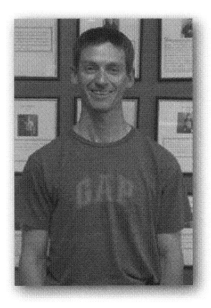

"Prior to my PT at Professional Physical Therapy and Sports Medicine, Inc., I had very limited range of motion in my right shoulder and at times severe or continuous throbbing in my shoulder. It was difficult to sleep at night, particularly on my right side, and I would have pain and numbness in my shoulder and arm if I moved my right arm too quickly. It was difficult to reach above my shoulders, behind my back, and across my body. Even the simple tasks of showering, tucking in my shirt, and reaching in my back pocket were challenging. I was diagnosed with "frozen shoulder" at Professional Physical Therapy and Sports Medicine. The staff was friendly, patient, and dedicated to getting me back to normal. I worked with several of the staff throughout my PT and was comfortable working with them all and appreciated their dedication and professionalism. I am now able to use my right shoulder to do more everyday tasks with no pain. My range of motion has significantly improved. My time here has helped resolve my limited motion, and the atmosphere has been relaxing, and I would recommend the facility to others."

—Walter Eaton

MY PHYSICAL THERAPY STORY

Maureen Doherty

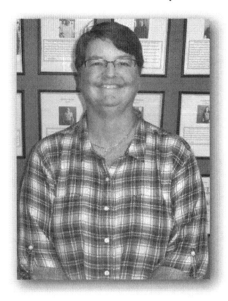

"I am a return client. Every two years I arrive back to have PT. The staff is very pleasant to work with, and they are very knowledgeable with the exercises that they ask you to do. I had a meniscus repair and the instability of my knee and muscle weakness were concerning to me because I work with small special needs children. Working with Sue, Amber, and Dr. Raybuck to build it up to have the strength, and the great care and compassion they all have for their clients helped me a lot. I will keep their phone number for future needs. Thanks to all of you."

—Maureen Doherty

MY PHYSICAL THERAPY STORY

Robin Holland

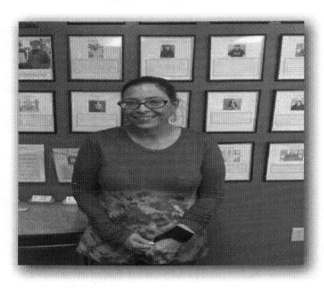

"I hurt my right shoulder while on vacation and was diagnosed with bursitis. The pain was extraordinary and I found myself in a sling. It was recommended to me that I start PT. There are few choices in town but I had heard great things about Pro PT and Sports Medicine. I called and was immediately given an appointment. I was initially assessed by Dr. Raybuck. Honestly, until I saw her I didn't even realize how impeded my range of motion was. I left that first day with a month's worth of appointments at just the time that worked with my busy schedule. I worked with both Sue and Amber, who not only are top notch at what they do, but are incredibly nice people. They explained things in a very easy to understand fashion and actually handed out pictures to make the exercises easier to understand. I will miss all the wonderful people at Pro PT!"

—Robin Holland

MY PHYSICAL THERAPY STORY

Tom Walczak

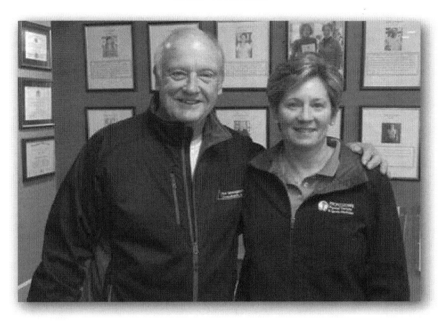

"The first day I came into PT I was using crutches. The IT band on my right upper leg was hurting tremendously. The bursa sac was on fire, and quite honestly I was scared. I asked myself what caused this problem and what would make it go away. I met with Dr. Raybuck and she explained everything in a way that I understood. This condition had developed over time without an accident or any main event. Dr. Raybuck laid out a plan, and Sue and Amber were excellent with their communication and execution. Today I have a home program that I will continue to do. My pain is gone except for rare moments. Thanks really doesn't say enough. Thank you!

—Tom Walczak

MY PHYSICAL THERAPY STORY

Dorothy Diskin

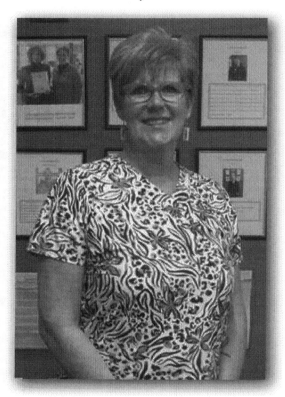

"I had just finished with a long-term injury (or at least what I considered long term). I had a surgical repair of a torn labrum in the hip and was out of work for ten weeks. Shortly after returning to my "normal" activities, I injured the knee on the opposite side. I had very little FMLA left and was in a panic. Fortunately, the MRI revealed that the knee was not a surgical issue and could be dealt with in PT. The first appointment I had with Dr. Raybuck gave me great hope as to what we could accomplish. She and her staff (Amber and Sue) were also amazing—always supportive and offering suggestions as well as challenging me to increase my strength.

Every person I encountered during my visits at Professional PT, both staff and fellow patients, were amazing. Also, the front office staff would greet me warmly and with a smile. I am now back to my normal activities with the outstanding help and support of Dr. Raybuck and her staff! Thank you to everyone."

—Dorothy Diskin

Regina Chambers

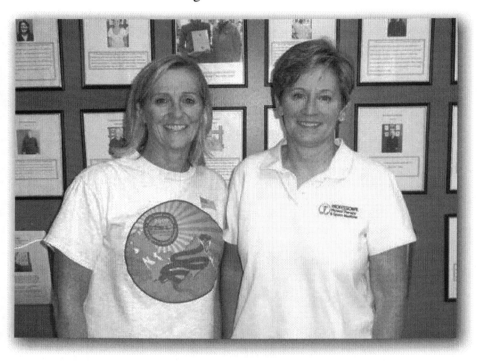

"Seeing an ad in the newspaper for a free back screening and taking the call to action and making an appointment with Dr. Raybuck was life changing. After living with back pain for over a year and missing triathlon training, I was skeptical I would ever be pain-free. With Dr. Raybuck's expertise and knowledge, I am back to training regularly, working as an occupational therapist in the school system...all PAIN-FREE! I can now complete long bike rides, hike, and play golf. The only problem I have now is that I don't have any excuses for a poor golf game!"

—Regina Chambers

MY PHYSICAL THERAPY STORY

Ron Lane

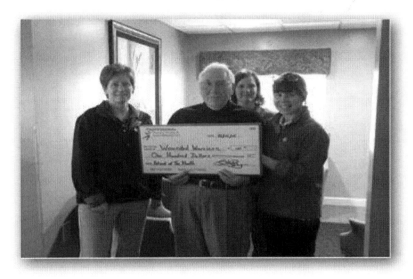

"There was no precipitating event; just one day lifting my head resulted in severe tingling pain down my right arm and into my fingers. If I kept looking up, pain would extend down my right side. My neck and shoulder muscles were tight, but this wasn't usual for me (bad posture and computer/reading hunch). It was, however, affecting my ability to drive. When the problem didn't resolve itself with some heat, I went to the doctor, who diagnosed a pinched nerve and prescribed muscle relaxants. When this didn't work, he sent me for x-rays of my neck, followed by an MRI. It turned out I had problems with my C6 vertebra, and that was the source of the pinching. Before prescribing surgery, the neurologist thought it wouldn't hurt to try physical therapy. Enter Dr. Raybuck and her crew of happy warriors.

During our initial consultation Dr. Raybuck observed that not only didn't I lift my head, but I also walked bent over like an old man (I am an old man, but still…). Undaunted by the challenge, however, she prescribed a course of therapy for her skilled staff to employ in returning me to some semblance of my former self. For many weeks they cheerfully guided me through many exercises designed to strengthen my muscles, even gleefully, I believe, ending each session by stretching my neck with their medieval traction device (I'm sure I'm at least four inches taller than when I started).

Now that I'm a graduate of Professional Physical Therapy, I can report that there is no more pain, my neck is probably 98 percent of normal, and my posture is 110 percent of what it was. Thank you, Dr. Raybuck and all your staff, especially Susan, for a wonderful experience. Good people doing good work. Blessed be."

—Ron Lane

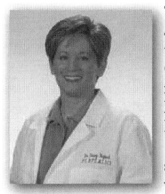

Dr. Stacey Raybuck Schatz, DPT, MS, OCS, has been providing physical therapy in clinical settings for thirty years. Concentrating in orthopedics and sports medicine, she owns and directs Professional Physical Therapy and Sports Medicine in Franklin, Massachusetts.

As a board-certified orthopedic clinical specialist, Dr. Raybuck Schatz has treated a wide range of patients, including athletes of all levels and non-athletes of various ages.

Her current clients are other healthcare providers across the nation, including clinicians for professional teams and for hospital or rehabilitation facilities. Alongside other providers, Dr. Raybuck Schatz advocates for choice-of-provider legislation and for policies that improve consumer protections.

Dr. Raybuck Schatz earned a bachelor's degree from the University of Massachusetts and master's and doctoral degrees from the Institute of Health Professions. She is a longtime member of the American Physical Therapy Association.

Made in the USA
Lexington, KY
25 November 2019